PCOS DIET COOKBOOK FOR NEWLY DIAGNOSED

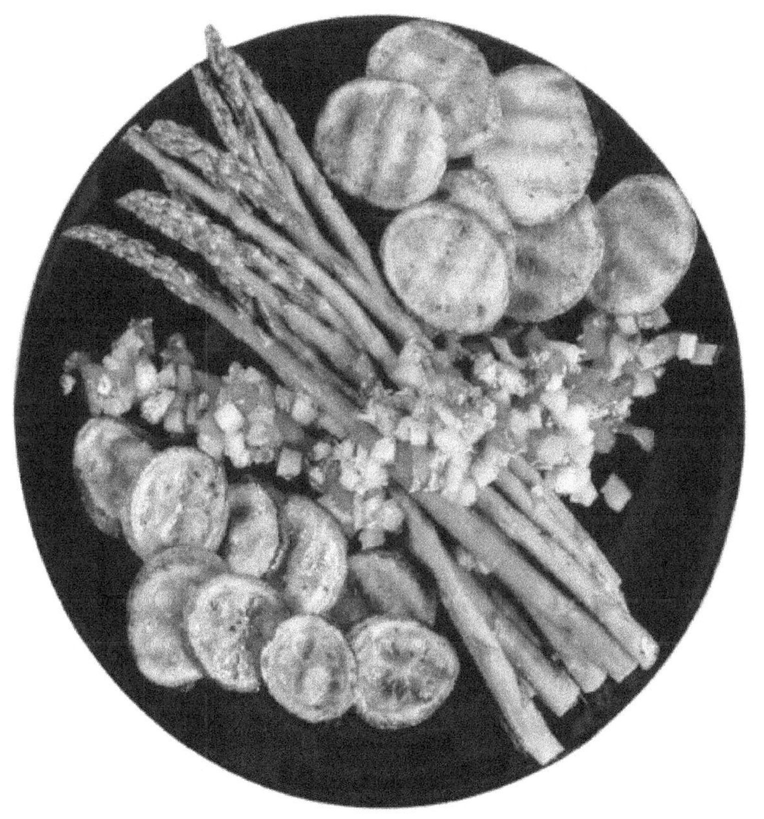

LYSANDRA QUINN

DISCLAIMER

The content within this book reflects my thoughts, experiences, and beliefs. It is meant for informational and entertainment purposes. While I have taken great care to provide accurate information, I cannot guarantee the absolute correctness or applicability of the content to every individual or situation. Please consult with relevant professionals for advice specific to your needs.

Contact the Author

Thank you for reading my book! I would love to hear from you, whether you have feedback, questions, or just want to share your thoughts. Your feedback means a lot to me and helps me improve as a writer.

Please don't hesitate to reach out to me through

contactmelysandraquinn@gmail.com

I look forward to connecting with my readers and appreciate your support in this literary journey. Your thoughts and comments are valuable to me.

TABLE OF CONTENTS

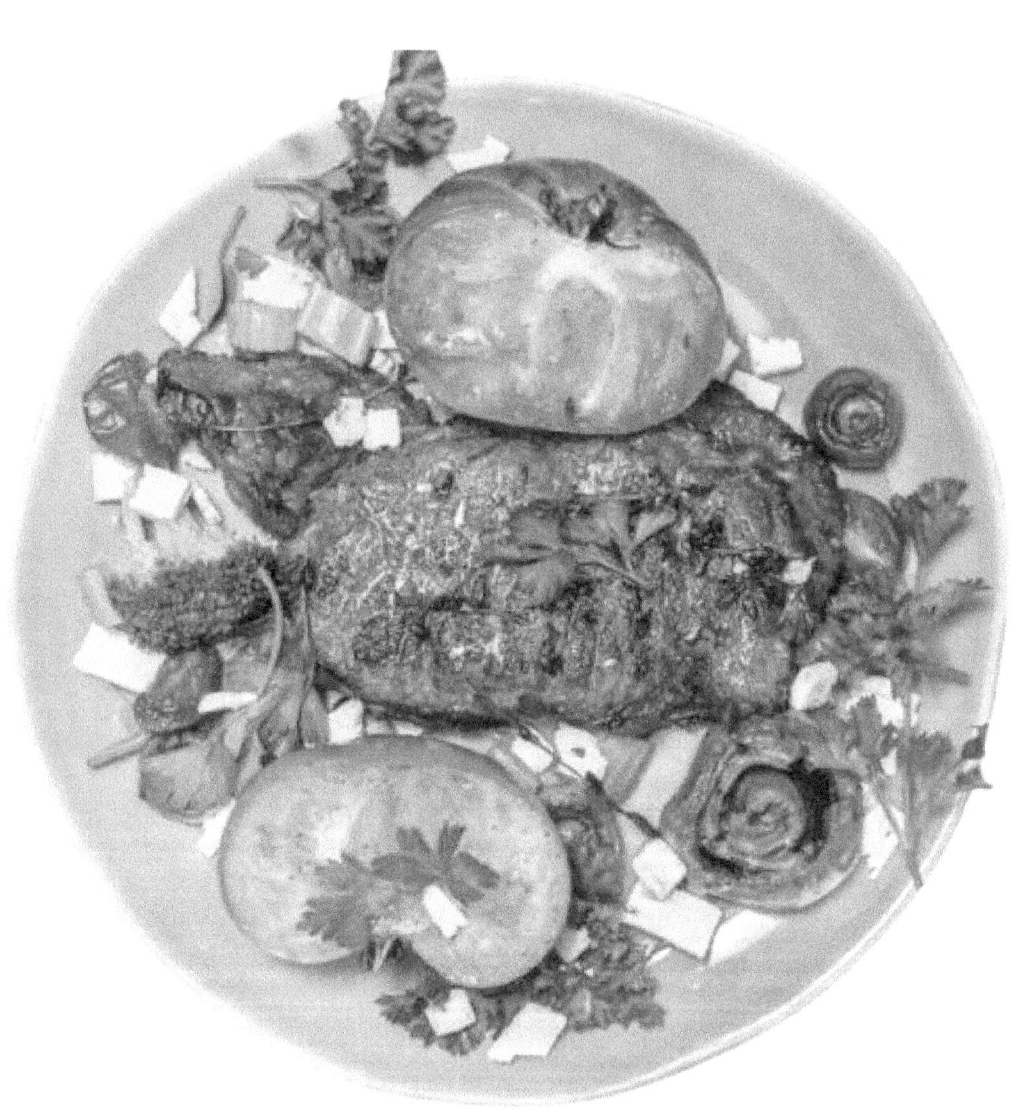

INTRODUCTION

In the quiet corners of our lives, where challenges lurk and shadows cast doubt, there exists a journey that many women embark upon, a journey that often starts with a diagnosis: Polycystic Ovary Syndrome (PCOS). It was in the hushed whispers of this diagnosis that I found myself weaving a tapestry of hope and healing for my dear friend Sophie. Her story, much like the stories of countless others, is a testament to the resilience of the human spirit and the transformative power of a well-crafted recipe.

Let me take you back to the time when Sophie and I first crossed paths, bound by the common thread of friendship. As a dedicated dietitian, my days were filled with the pursuit of knowledge, especially when it came to unravelling the mysteries of PCOS. Sophie, newly diagnosed and grappling with the challenges it presented, found herself lost in a maze of conflicting advice and disappointing outcomes from various cookbooks. Each attempt to find solace in the pages of those cookbooks felt like another step into a foggy abyss.

The journey began when Sophie approached me, her eyes reflecting a mixture of frustration and longing for a glimmer of hope. She had navigated through cookbook after cookbook, each promising a solution to her PCOS-related struggles. Yet, the results were elusive, and the frustration etched on her face mirrored the silent battles fought by countless women facing this condition.

As a friend and a dietician, I couldn't stand idly by. I had spent years immersed in the world of PCOS research, studying the intricate dance between hormones and nutrition, and I decided it was time to share the fruits of that Labor with Sophie. The exchange of recipes marked the beginning of a culinary journey that would soon blossom into a life-changing experience.

The transformation in Sophie was not immediate, but it was profound. Slowly but surely, the carefully curated recipes began to cast a warm light into the shadows of her PCOS journey. It wasn't just about what was on her plate; it was about the nourishment that seeped into her body, the healing whispers of ingredients working in harmony to restore balance.

It took a couple of years, but the changes in Sophie were undeniable. Her energy levels surged, the cloud of fatigue lifted, and the weight that had become a burdensome companion began to melt away. Witnessing her journey was nothing short of inspiring, and it was then that the seeds of this cookbook were sown.

As I pen down these words, it is with a heart full of empathy and a burning desire to extend a lifeline to every woman grappling with PCOS. This cookbook is not just a collection of recipes; it is a lifeline, a beacon of hope that pierces through the darkness of uncertainty. It's a symphony of Flavors and nutrients, crafted with love and precision to empower you on your journey towards wellness.

Now, I invite you to embark on this culinary odyssey with me. But before you turn the pages and delve into the recipes that have transformed lives, let me ask you this: Have you ever felt the frustration of flipping through cookbook after cookbook, only to be met with disappointment and despair? Can you imagine the joy of discovering recipes that not only tantalize your taste buds but also heal your body from within?

Picture this: a warm kitchen bathed in soft light, the aroma of wholesome ingredients wafting through the air, and the promise of a brighter, healthier future on your plate. As you leaf through these pages, let the stories of Sophie and countless others resonate with you. Let the shared triumphs and victories become a source of inspiration, a reminder that you are not alone on this journey.

Are you ready to embark on a culinary adventure that transcends the boundaries of a mere cookbook? This is not just about food; it's about reclaiming your vitality, embracing your body, and savouring the joy of a life well-nourished. Let the pages that follow be a testament to the transformative power of a simple recipe, and may this cookbook be the compass that guides you towards a healthier, happier you.

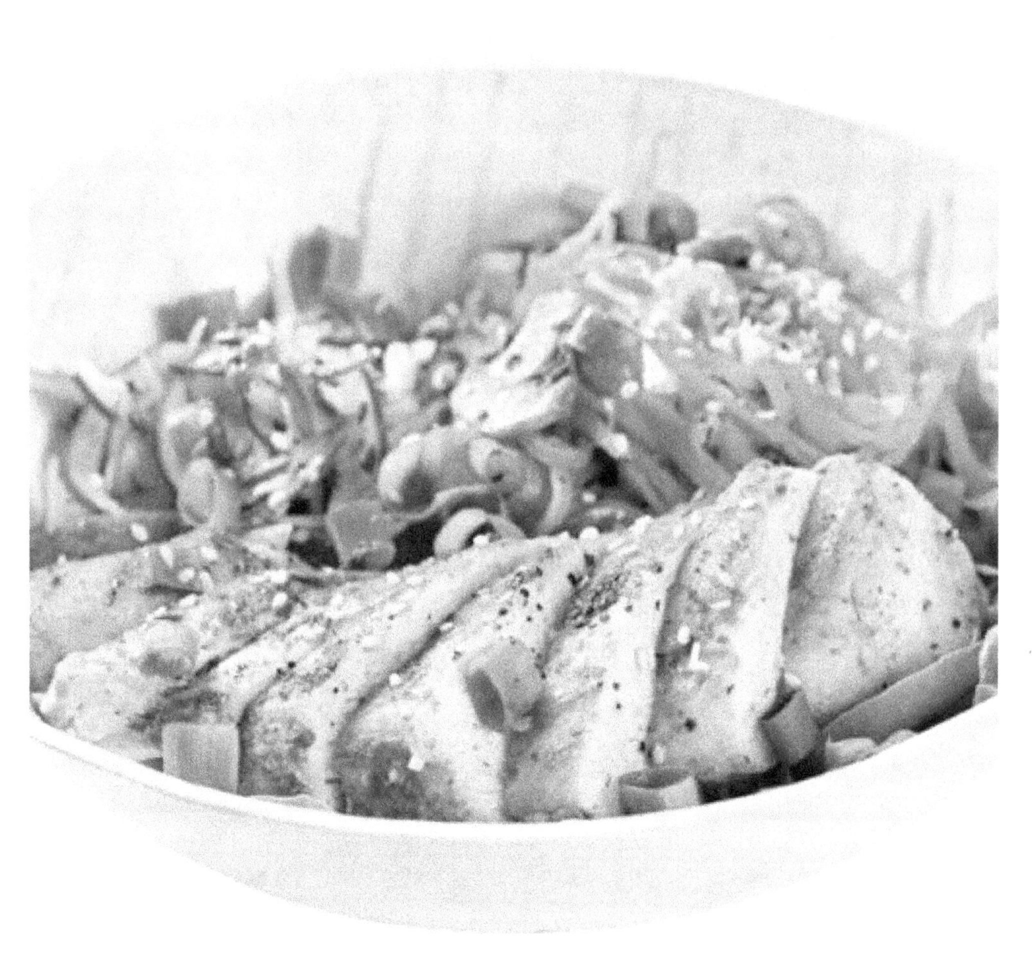

CHAPTER 1

PCOS BASICS

PCOS, or Polycystic Ovary Syndrome, is a common hormonal disorder that affects individuals with ovaries, typically during their reproductive years. It is characterized by a variety of symptoms and can have implications for both reproductive and overall health.

Common Symptoms:

Irregular Menstrual Cycles: Women with PCOS often experience irregular periods, which can manifest as infrequent or prolonged menstrual cycles.

Ovulatory Dysfunction: PCOS can disrupt the normal ovulation process, leading to irregular or absent ovulation, which may contribute to fertility issues.

Hyperandrogenism: Elevated levels of androgens (male hormones) in women can result in symptoms such as acne, excessive facial or body hair (hirsutism), and male-pattern baldness.

Polycystic Ovaries: Despite the name, not all women with PCOS have cysts on their ovaries. However, an ultrasound may reveal enlarged ovaries with small, fluid-filled sacs (follicles) surrounding the eggs.

Insulin Resistance: Many individuals with PCOS have insulin resistance, which can lead to elevated insulin levels. This can contribute to weight gain and increase the risk of type 2 diabetes.

Weight Gain: PCOS is associated with weight gain, and individuals with excess weight may be more prone to developing the syndrome.

Causes and Risk Factors:

The exact cause of PCOS is not fully understood, but it is believed to involve a combination of genetic and environmental factors. Some key factors include:

Genetics: There appears to be a genetic component, as women with a family history of PCOS are at a higher risk.

Insulin Resistance: Insulin resistance, a condition where the body's cells do not respond effectively to insulin, is a common factor in PCOS. This can lead to increased insulin levels and elevated androgen production.

Hormonal Imbalance: PCOS is characterized by an imbalance in reproductive hormones, including elevated levels of luteinizing hormone (LH) and increased production of androgens.

Inflammation: Chronic low-grade inflammation may play a role in the development of PCOS.

Lifestyle Factors: Poor diet, lack of physical activity, and excess weight can contribute to the development and exacerbation of PCOS symptoms.

Management and Treatment:

While PCOS cannot be cured, its symptoms can be managed through lifestyle changes, medications, and, in some cases, fertility treatments. Lifestyle modifications, such as a healthy diet, regular exercise, and weight management, are often recommended to improve insulin sensitivity and hormonal balance.

CHAPTER 2

PCOS-FRIENDLY FOODS

Polycystic Ovary Syndrome (PCOS) management often involves adopting a balanced and PCOS-friendly diet. Choosing the right foods can help regulate hormones, manage weight, and improve overall health. Here's an overview of PCOS-friendly foods:

High-Fiber Foods: Incorporate whole grains, fruits, vegetables, and legumes into your diet. High-fiber foods can help regulate blood sugar levels and improve insulin sensitivity, which is crucial for individuals with PCOS.

Lean Proteins: Opt for lean protein sources such as poultry, fish, tofu, legumes, and low-fat dairy. Protein-rich foods help with satiety, weight management, and muscle maintenance.

Healthy Fats: Include sources of healthy fats, such as avocados, nuts, seeds, and olive oil. These fats are important for hormone production and can contribute to a feeling of fullness.

Low-Glycemic Index (GI) Foods: Choose carbohydrates with a low glycemic index to prevent rapid spikes in blood sugar. Examples include sweet potatoes, quinoa, and whole grains.

Anti-Inflammatory Foods: Include foods with anti-inflammatory properties, such as fatty fish (like salmon), turmeric, ginger, and green leafy vegetables. Chronic inflammation is associated with PCOS, and these foods may help manage it.

Foods Rich in Omega-3 Fatty Acids: Omega-3 fatty acids, found in fish, flaxseeds, and chia seeds, have anti-inflammatory effects and may support hormonal balance.

Importance of Balanced Nutrition:

Maintaining a balanced diet is crucial for managing PCOS symptoms and promoting overall well-being. Here's why balanced nutrition is important for individuals with PCOS:

Blood Sugar Control: Balanced meals and snacks can help regulate blood sugar levels, reducing insulin resistance associated with PCOS.

Hormonal Balance: Nutrient-dense foods support hormonal balance, addressing imbalances commonly seen in PCOS.

Weight Management: A balanced diet, coupled with appropriate portion control, can contribute to weight management, which is often a key aspect of PCOS management.

Energy Levels: Proper nutrition ensures an adequate intake of vitamins and minerals, supporting energy levels and reducing fatigue.

Reduced Inflammation: Anti-inflammatory foods can help mitigate chronic inflammation associated with PCOS.

Grocery Shopping Tips:

Focus on Fresh Produce: Fill your cart with a variety of colorful fruits and vegetables. These nutrient-dense foods are rich in vitamins, minerals, and antioxidants.

Choose Whole Grains: opt for whole grains like brown rice, quinoa, oats, and whole wheat bread. These provide fiber and have a lower glycemic index.

Select Lean Proteins: Choose lean sources of protein, such as skinless poultry, fish, tofu, legumes, and low-fat dairy products.

Incorporate Healthy Fats: Include avocados, nuts, seeds, and olive oil in your shopping list to incorporate healthy fats into your diet.

Read Labels: Pay attention to food labels to avoid processed foods with added sugars and unhealthy fats. Choose minimally processed, whole foods whenever possible.

Stay Hydrated: Water is essential for overall health. Limit sugary drinks and opt for water, herbal teas, or infused water.

CHAPTER 1

BREAKFAST RECIPES

Quinoa Breakfast Bowl:

Cooking Time: 15 minutes

Servings: 2

Ingredients:

- 1 cup cooked quinoa
- 1/2 cup berries (e.g., blueberries, strawberries)
- 2 tablespoons chopped nuts (e.g., almonds, walnuts)
- 1 tablespoon chia seeds
- Greek yogurt (optional)

Instructions:

1. Mix cooked quinoa with berries, nuts, and chia seeds.
2. Top with a dollop of Greek yogurt if desired.

Nutritional Information (per serving):

Calories: 300, Carbs: 45g, Protein: 10g, Fat: 10g, Fiber: 8g

Omelet with Vegetables:

Cooking Time: 10 minutes

Servings: 1

Ingredients:

- 2 eggs
- 1/2 cup chopped vegetables (bell peppers, spinach, tomatoes)
- 1 tablespoon olive oil
- Salt and pepper to taste

Instructions:

1. Whisk eggs and mix in chopped vegetables.
2. Heat olive oil in a pan, pour in the egg mixture, and cook until set.

Nutritional Information:

Calories: 280, Carbs: 10g, Protein: 15g, Fat: 20g, Fiber: 3g

Greek Yogurt Parfait:

Preparation Time: 5 minutes

Servings: 1

Ingredients:

- 1 cup Greek yogurt
- 1/2 cup mixed berries
- 2 tablespoons granola
- 1 tablespoon honey

Instructions:

1. Layer Greek yogurt with berries and granola.
2. Drizzle honey on top.

Nutritional Information:

Calories: 280, Carbs: 35g, Protein: 15g, Fat: 8g, Fiber: 4g

Sweet Potato Toast with Avocado:

Cooking Time: 20 minutes

Servings: 2

Ingredients:

- 1 large, sweet potato, sliced.
- 1 avocado, mashed.
- Cherry tomatoes, sliced.
- Salt and pepper to taste

Instructions:

1. Toast sweet potato slices until cooked.
2. Spread mashed avocado on top and add sliced cherry tomatoes.

Nutritional Information (per serving):

Calories: 220, Carbs: 30g, Protein: 3g, Fat: 12g, Fiber: 7g

Chia Seed Pudding:

Preparation Time: 5 minutes (plus chilling time)

Servings: 2

Ingredients:

- 1/4 cup chia seeds
- 1 cup almond milk
- 1/2 teaspoon vanilla extract
- Sliced strawberries and almonds for topping

Instructions:

1. Mix chia seeds, almond milk, and vanilla extract. Refrigerate for a few hours or overnight.
2. Top with sliced strawberries and almonds before serving.

Nutritional Information (per serving):

Calories: 180, Carbs: 20g, Protein: 6g, Fat: 9g, Fiber: 10g

Spinach and Feta Egg Muffins:

Cooking Time: 25 minutes

Servings: 4

Ingredients:

- 6 eggs
- 1 cup chopped spinach.
- 1/2 cup crumbled feta cheese
- Salt and pepper to taste

Instructions:

1. Preheat the oven. Whisk eggs and mix in spinach, feta, salt, and pepper.
2. Pour into muffin cups and bake until set.

Nutritional Information (per serving):

Calories: 150, Carbs: 2g, Protein: 12g, Fat: 10g, Fiber: 1g

Berry Smoothie Bowl:

Preparation Time: 10 minutes

Servings: 1

Ingredients:

- 1 cup mixed berries (frozen or fresh)
- 1/2 banana
- 1/2 cup Greek yogurt
- 1 tablespoon almond butter
- 1/4 cup granola

Instructions:

1. Blend berries, banana, Greek yogurt, and almond butter until smooth.
2. Pour into a bowl and top with granola.

Nutritional Information:

Calories: 320, Carbs: 40g, Protein: 15g, Fat: 12g. Fiber: 6g

Avocado and Tomato Breakfast Wrap:

Preparation Time: 15 minutes

Servings: 1

Ingredients:

- 1 whole-grain tortilla
- 1/2 avocado, sliced.
- Cherry tomatoes, sliced.
- Scrambled eggs
- Salsa (optional)

Instructions:

1. Fill the tortilla with sliced avocado, tomatoes, and scrambled eggs.
2. Add salsa if desired, then fold into a wrap.

Nutritional Information:

Calories: 350, Carbs: 30g, Protein: 15g, Fat: 18g, Fiber: 8g

Cottage Cheese and Pineapple Bowl:

Preparation Time: 5 minutes

Servings: 1

Ingredients:

- 1 cup low-fat cottage cheese
- 1/2 cup fresh pineapple chunks
- 1 tablespoon flaxseeds

Instructions:

1. Combine cottage cheese with pineapple chunks.
2. Sprinkle flaxseeds on top.

Nutritional Information:

Calories: 280, Carbs: 25g, Protein: 30g, Fat: 8g, Fiber: 3g

Whole Grain Pancakes with Berries:

Cooking Time: 15 minutes

Servings: 2

Ingredients:

- 1 cup whole grain pancake mix
- 1 cup almond milk
- 1 egg
- Mixed berries for topping

Instructions:

1. Mix pancake mix, almond milk, and egg until smooth.
2. Cook pancakes on a griddle and top with mixed berries.

Nutritional Information (per serving):

Calories: 250, Carbs: 40g, Protein: 8g, Fat: 6g, Fiber: 5g

CHAPTER 2

LUNCH RECIPES

Grilled Chicken Salad:

Cooking Time: 20 minutes

Servings: 2

Ingredients:

- 2 boneless, skinless chicken breasts
- Mixed salad greens
- Cherry tomatoes, halved.
- Cucumber, sliced.
- Avocado, diced.

Instructions:

1. Grill chicken until cooked through.
2. Slice the chicken and arrange it on a bed of salad greens with tomatoes, cucumber, and avocado.

Nutritional Information (per serving):

Calories: 300, Carbs: 15g, Protein: 30g, Fat: 15g, Fiber: 8g

Quinoa and Vegetable Stir-Fry:

Cooking Time: 25 minutes

Servings: 4

Ingredients:

- 1 cup quinoa, cooked.
- Mixed vegetables (broccoli, bell peppers, carrots)
- Tofu or chicken, cubed.
- Low-sodium soy sauce

Instructions:

1. Stir-fry tofu or chicken with vegetables until cooked.
2. Mix in cooked quinoa and add soy sauce to taste.

Nutritional Information (per serving):

Calories: 320, Carbs: 45g, Protein: 15g, Fat: 10g, Fiber: 7g

Salmon and Asparagus Foil Packets:

Cooking Time: 20 minutes

Servings: 2

Ingredients:

- 2 salmon fillets
- Asparagus spears
- Lemon slices
- Olive oil, salt, and pepper

Instructions:

1. Place salmon and asparagus on a foil sheet.
2. Drizzle with olive oil, add lemon slices, and season with salt and pepper. Seal into packets and bake.

Nutritional Information (per serving):

Calories: 350, Carbs: 10g, Protein: 30g, Fat: 20g, Fiber: 5g

Turkey and Veggie Lettuce Wraps:

Cooking Time: 15 minutes

Servings: 3

Ingredients:

- Ground turkey
- Lettuce leaves
- Onion, diced.
- Bell peppers, sliced.
- Taco seasoning

Instructions:

1. Cook ground turkey with diced onions and sliced bell peppers.
2. Season with taco seasoning and serve in lettuce wraps.

Nutritional Information (per serving):

Calories: 250, Carbs: 10g, Protein: 20g, Fat: 15g, Fiber: 3g

Mediterranean Chickpea Salad:

Preparation Time: 15 minutes

Servings: 4

Ingredients:

- 1 can chickpeas, drained
- Cherry tomatoes, halved.
- Cucumber, diced.
- Feta cheese, crumbled.
- Kalamata olives

Instructions:

1. Combine chickpeas, tomatoes, cucumber, feta, and olives.
2. Drizzle with olive oil and toss to combine.

Nutritional Information (per serving):

Calories: 280, Carbs: 30g, Protein: 12g, Fat: 14g, Fiber: 8g

Vegetarian Quinoa Bowl:

Cooking Time: 25 minutes

Servings: 3

Ingredients:

- 1 cup quinoa, cooked.
- Black beans, drained
- Corn kernels
- Avocado, diced.
- Salsa and cilantro for topping

Instructions:

1. Mix cooked quinoa with black beans, corn, and diced avocado.
2. Top with salsa and cilantro.

Nutritional Information (per serving):

Calories: 320, Carbs: 50g, Protein: 10g, Fat: 10g, Fiber: 12g

Lemon Garlic Shrimp Pasta:

Cooking Time: 20 minutes

Servings: 2

Ingredients:

- Whole wheat pasta
- Shrimp peeled and deveined.
- Garlic, minced.
- Lemon juice and zest
- Spinach leaves

Instructions:

1. Cook pasta according to package instructions.
2. Sauté shrimp and garlic, add cooked pasta, lemon juice, and zest. Toss in spinach until wilted.

Nutritional Information (per serving):

Calories: 340, Carbs: 45g, Protein: 25g, Fat: 8g, Fiber: 7g

Egg and Vegetable Stir-Fried Brown Rice:

Cooking Time: 15 minutes

Servings: 2

Ingredients:

- Brown rice, cooked.
- Eggs, beaten.
- Mixed vegetables (broccoli, carrots, peas)
- Low-sodium soy sauce

Instructions:

1. Stir-fry mixed vegetables, add beaten eggs, and scramble.
2. Mix in cooked brown rice and add soy sauce to taste.

Nutritional Information (per serving):

Calories: 300, Carbs: 50g, Protein: 15g, Fat: 8g, Fiber: 6g

Sweet Potato and Chickpea Buddha Bowl:

Cooking Time: 30 minutes

Servings: 2

Ingredients:

- Sweet potatoes, cubed.
- Chickpeas, drained and rinsed.
- Quinoa, cooked.
- Avocado, sliced.
- Tahini dressing

Instructions:

1. Roast sweet potatoes and chickpeas until golden.
2. Assemble bowls with quinoa, roasted veggies, and sliced avocado. Drizzle with tahini dressing.

Nutritional Information (per serving):

Calories: 380, Carbs: 50g, Protein: 12g, Fat: 18g, Fiber: 10g

Turkey and Vegetable Stuffed Bell Peppers:

Cooking Time: 40 minutes

Servings: 4

Ingredients:

- Ground turkey
- Quinoa, cooked.
- Bell peppers, halved.
- Tomato sauce
- Mozzarella cheese, shredded.

Instructions:

1. Brown ground turkey, mix with cooked quinoa.
2. Stuff bell peppers with the turkey-quinoa mixture, top with tomato sauce and cheese. Bake until peppers are tender.

Nutritional Information (per serving):

Calories: 320, Carbs: 25g, Protein: 25g, Fat: 15g, Fiber: 6g

CHAPTER 3

DINNER RECIPES

Baked Lemon Herb Chicken:

Cooking Time: 30 minutes

Servings: 2

Ingredients:

- 2 boneless, skinless chicken breasts
- Lemon juice, olive oil, garlic, thyme, rosemary
- Salt and pepper to taste

Instructions:

1. Marinate chicken in a mixture of lemon juice, olive oil, garlic, thyme, rosemary, salt, and pepper.
2. Bake until the chicken is cooked through.

Nutritional Information (per serving):

Calories: 300, Carbs: 2g, Protein: 30g, Fat: 20g, Fiber: 1g

Vegetarian Lentil Soup:

Cooking Time: 40 minutes

Servings: 4

Ingredients:

- 1 cup dry lentils
- Vegetables (carrots, celery, onions)
- Vegetable broth, garlic, cumin, coriander

Instructions:

1. Sauté vegetables, add lentils, and then pour in vegetable broth.
2. Season with garlic, cumin, and coriander. Simmer until lentils are tender.

Nutritional Information (per serving):

Calories: 250, Carbs: 40g, Protein: 15g, Fat: 2g, Fiber: 15g

Grilled Salmon with Broccoli and Quinoa:

Cooking Time: 25 minutes

Servings: 2

Ingredients:

- Salmon fillets
- Broccoli florets
- Quinoa, cooked.
- Olive oil, lemon juice, garlic

Instructions:

1. Grill salmon and steamed broccoli.
2. Serve over a bed of cooked quinoa. Drizzle with olive oil, lemon juice, and minced garlic.

Nutritional Information (per serving):

Calories: 380, Carbs: 30g, Protein: 30g, Fat: 18g, Fiber: 6g

Turkey and Vegetable Stir-Fry with Brown Rice:

Cooking Time: 20 minutes

Servings: 3

Ingredients:

- Ground turkey
- Mixed vegetables (bell peppers, broccoli, carrots)
- Brown rice, cooked.
- Low-sodium soy sauce, ginger, garlic

Instructions:

1. Stir-fry ground turkey and mixed vegetables.
2. Add cooked brown rice and season with low-sodium soy sauce, ginger, and garlic.

Nutritional Information (per serving):

Calories: 320, Carbs: 40g, Protein: 20g, Fat: 10g, Fiber: 6g

Eggplant and Chickpea Curry:

Cooking Time: 35 minutes

Servings: 4

Ingredients:

- Eggplant, diced.
- Chickpeas, drained and rinsed.
- Onion, tomatoes, garlic, ginger
- Curry spices (turmeric, cumin, coriander)

Instructions:

1. Sauté onions, garlic, and ginger. Add diced eggplant and cook until tender.
2. Stir in chickpeas, tomatoes, and curry spices. Simmer until flavors meld.

Nutritional Information (per serving):

Calories: 280, Carbs: 35g, Protein: 12g, Fat: 10g, Fiber: 12g

Cauliflower Fried Rice with Shrimp:

Cooking Time: 25 minutes

Servings: 3

Ingredients:

- Cauliflower rice
- Shrimp peeled and deveined.
- Mixed vegetables (peas, carrots, corn)
- Soy sauce, sesame oil, ginger

Instructions:

1. Stir-fry shrimp and mixed vegetables. Add cauliflower rice.
2. Season with soy sauce, sesame oil, and ginger.

Nutritional Information (per serving):

Calories: 250, Carbs: 20g, Protein: 25g, Fat: 10g, Fiber: 8g

Spaghetti Squash with Turkey Bolognese:

Cooking Time: 45 minutes

Servings: 2

Ingredients:

- Spaghetti squash
- Ground turkey
- Tomato sauce, onions, garlic, Italian herbs

Instructions:

1. Roast spaghetti squash and scrape out the strands.
2. In a separate pan, cook ground turkey with onions, garlic, tomato sauce, and Italian herbs. Serve over spaghetti squash.

Nutritional Information (per serving):

Calories: 320, Carbs: 30g, Protein: 25g, Fat: 12g, Fiber: 8g

Stuffed Bell Peppers with Quinoa and Black Beans:

Cooking Time: 40 minutes

Servings: 4

Ingredients:

- Bell peppers
- Quinoa, cooked.
- Black beans, drained and rinsed.
- Onion, tomatoes, corn

Instructions:

1. Cut bell peppers in half and remove seeds.
2. Mix cooked quinoa with black beans, diced tomatoes, and corn. Stuff the bell peppers and bake.

Nutritional Information (per serving):

Calories: 280, Carbs: 45g, Protein: 15g, Fat: 6g, Fiber: 10g

Lemon Garlic Shrimp Zoodle Bowl:

Cooking Time: 20 minutes

Servings: 2

Ingredients:

- Shrimp, peeled and deveined.
- Zucchini noodles (zoodles)
- Lemon juice, garlic, olive oil, cherry tomatoes

Instructions:

1. Sauté shrimp in olive oil with garlic and cherry tomatoes.
2. Toss with zucchini noodles and lemon juice until heated through.

Nutritional Information (per serving):

Calories: 280, Carbs: 15g, Protein: 25g, Fat: 15g, Fiber: 5g

Chickpea and Spinach Curry:

Cooking Time: 30 minutes

Servings: 3

Ingredients:

- Chickpeas, drained and rinsed.
- Fresh spinach
- Onion, tomatoes, garlic, ginger
- Curry spices (cumin, coriander, turmeric)

Instructions:

1. Sauté onions, garlic, and ginger. Add chickpeas, tomatoes, and curry spices.
2. Once chickpeas are tender, stir in fresh spinach until wilted.

Nutritional Information (per serving):

Calories: 260, Carbs: 40g, Protein: 15g, Fat: 8g, Fiber: 12g

CHAPTER 4

SNACKS AND SIDES

Greek Yogurt and Berry Parfait:

Preparation Time: 5 minutes

Servings: 1

Ingredients:

- 1 cup Greek yogurt
- Mixed berries (blueberries, strawberries)
- Granola
- Honey (optional)

Instructions:

1. Layer Greek yogurt with mixed berries and granola.
2. Drizzle with honey if desired.

Nutritional Information (per serving):

Calories: 250, Carbs: 30g, Protein: 15g, Fat: 8g, Fiber: 4g

Cucumber and Hummus Slices:

Preparation Time: 10 minutes

Servings: 2

Ingredients:

- Cucumber, sliced.
- Hummus
- Cherry tomatoes, halved.

Instructions:

1. Slice cucumber and spread hummus on each slice.
2. Top with halved cherry tomatoes.

Nutritional Information (per serving):

Calories: 120, Carbs: 15g, Protein: 5g, Fat: 6g, Fiber: 4g

Roasted Chickpeas:

Preparation Time: 40 minutes

Servings: 4

Ingredients:

- 2 cans chickpeas, drained and rinsed.
- Olive oil, paprika, cumin, salt

Instructions:

1. Toss chickpeas in olive oil and spices.
2. Roast in the oven until crispy.

Nutritional Information (per serving):

Calories: 180, Carbs: 30g, Protein: 10g, Fat: 4g, Fiber: 8g

Avocado and Tomato Salsa:

Preparation Time: 15 minutes

Servings: 3

Ingredients:

- 2 avocados, diced.
- Tomatoes, diced.
- Red onion finely chopped.
- Cilantro, chopped.
- Lime juice, salt, pepper

Instructions:

1. Combine diced avocados, tomatoes, red onion, and cilantro.
2. Squeeze lime juice and season with salt and pepper.

Nutritional Information (per serving):

Calories: 180, Carbs: 12g, Protein: 3g, Fat: 15g, Fiber: 8g

Sweet Potato Chips:

Cooking Time: 25 minutes

Servings: 2

Ingredients:

- Sweet potatoes thinly sliced.
- Olive oil, paprika, salt

Instructions:

1. Toss sweet potato slices in olive oil and seasonings.
2. Bake until crispy.

Nutritional Information (per serving):

Calories: 120, Carbs: 20g, Protein: 2g, Fat: 4g, Fiber: 3g

Edamame and Sea Salt:

Cooking Time: 5 minutes

Servings: 2

Ingredients:

- Edamame cooked and cooled.
- Sea salt

Instructions:

1. Sprinkle cooked edamame with sea salt.
2. Serve as a protein-rich snack.

Nutritional Information (per serving):

Calories: 120, Carbs: 10g, Protein: 11g, Fat: 4g, Fiber: 5g

Quinoa Salad with Veggies:

Preparation Time: 20 minutes

Servings: 3

Ingredients:

- 1 cup quinoa, cooked.
- Cherry tomatoes, cucumber, bell peppers
- Feta cheese, olives
- Olive oil, lemon juice, oregano

Instructions:

1. Mix cooked quinoa with chopped vegetables, feta, and olives.
2. Drizzle with olive oil, lemon juice, and sprinkle with oregano.

Nutritional Information (per serving):

Calories: 250, Carbs: 30g, Protein: 8g, Fat: 12g, Fiber: 5g

Almond and Berry Smoothie:

Preparation Time: 10 minutes

Servings: 1

Ingredients:

- 1 cup almond milk
- Mixed berries (strawberries, blueberries)
- Almond butter
- Greek yogurt (optional)

Instructions:

1. Blend almond milk, mixed berries, and a spoonful of almond butter.
2. Add Greek yogurt for creaminess if desired.

Nutritional Information (per serving):

Calories: 220, Carbs: 25g, Protein: 8g, Fat: 10g, Fiber: 5g

Caprese Skewers:

Preparation Time: 15 minutes

Servings: 4

Ingredients:

- Cherry tomatoes
- Mozzarella balls
- Basil leaves
- Balsamic glaze

Instructions:

1. Thread cherry tomatoes, mozzarella balls, and basil leaves onto skewers.
2. Drizzle with balsamic glaze before serving.

Nutritional Information (per serving):

Calories: 150, Carbs: 5g, Protein: 8g, Fat: 10g, Fiber: 1g

Apple Slices with Almond Butter:

Preparation Time: 5 minutes

Servings: 2

Ingredients:

- Apples, sliced.
- Almond butter
- Cinnamon (optional)

Instructions:

1. Spread almond butter on apple slices.
2. Sprinkle with cinnamon if desired.

Nutritional Information (per serving):

Calories: 180, Carbs: 20g, Protein: 4g, Fat: 10g, Fiber: 5g

CHAPTER 5

DESSERTS AND TREATS

Chia Seed Pudding with Berries:

Preparation Time: 5 minutes (plus chilling time)

Servings: 2

Ingredients:

- 1/4 cup chia seeds
- 1 cup almond milk
- 1/2 teaspoon vanilla extract
- Mixed berries for topping

Instructions:

1. Mix chia seeds, almond milk, and vanilla extract. Refrigerate for a few hours or overnight.
2. Top with mixed berries before serving.

Nutritional Information (per serving):

Calories: 180, Carbs: 20g, Protein: 6g, Fat: 9g, Fiber: 10g

Dark Chocolate Avocado Mousse:

Preparation Time: 15 minutes

Servings: 4

Ingredients:

- 2 ripe avocados
- 1/4 cup unsweetened cocoa powder
- 1/4 cup maple syrup
- 1 teaspoon vanilla extract

Instructions:

1. Blend avocados, cocoa powder, maple syrup, and vanilla extract until smooth.
2. Chill before serving.

Nutritional Information (per serving):

Calories: 200, Carbs: 20g, Protein: 3g, Fat: 15g, Fiber: 8g

Berry and Yogurt Parfait:

Preparation Time: 10 minutes

Servings: 2

Ingredients:

- Greek yogurt
- Mixed berries (strawberries, blueberries)
- Granola

Instructions:

1. Layer Greek yogurt with mixed berries and granola.
2. Repeat layers until the glass is filled.

Nutritional Information (per serving):

Calories: 250, Carbs: 30g, Protein: 15g, Fat: 8g, Fiber: 4g

Baked Apples with Cinnamon and Walnuts:

Cooking Time: 30 minutes

Servings: 2

Ingredients:

- 2 apples cored and sliced.
- Cinnamon
- Chopped walnuts.
- Maple syrup (optional)

Instructions:

1. Preheat the oven. Toss apple slices with cinnamon and walnuts.
2. Bake until apples are tender. Drizzle with maple syrup if desired.

Nutritional Information (per serving):

Calories: 180, Carbs: 30g, Protein: 2g, Fat: 8g, Fiber: 6g

Coconut and Almond Energy Bites:

Preparation Time: 15 minutes

Servings: 12

Ingredients:

- 1 cup unsweetened shredded coconut
- 1/2 cup almond flour
- 1/4 cup coconut oil, melted.
- 1/4 cup almond butter
- Vanilla extract, stevia (optional)

Instructions:

1. Mix shredded coconut, almond flour, melted coconut oil, almond butter, and vanilla extract.
2. Roll into bite-sized balls and chill before serving.

Nutritional Information (per serving - 2 bites):

Calories: 150, Carbs: 6g, Protein: 3g, Fat: 12g, Fiber: 3g

Frozen Banana Pops:

Preparation Time: 10 minutes (plus freezing time)

Servings: 4

Ingredients:

- Bananas peeled and halved.
- Greek yogurt
- Crushed nuts or shredded coconut (optional)

Instructions:

1. Dip banana halves in Greek yogurt and coat with crushed nuts or shredded coconut if desired.
2. Freeze until firm.

Nutritional Information (per serving):

Calories: 120, Carbs: 25g, Protein: 3g, Fat: 2g, Fiber: 3g

Protein-Packed Chocolate Smoothie Bowl:

Preparation Time: 10 minutes

Servings: 1

Ingredients:

- 1 scoop chocolate protein powder
- Frozen berries
- Almond milk
- Toppings: sliced almonds, chia seeds, shredded coconut

Instructions:

1. Blend protein powder, frozen berries, and almond milk until smooth.
2. Pour into a bowl and add your favorite toppings.

Nutritional Information (per serving):

Calories: 300, Carbs: 25g, Protein: 25g, Fat: 12g, Fiber: 8g

Ricotta and Berry Stuffed Crepes:

Cooking Time: 20 minutes

Servings: 3

Ingredients:

- Crepes (store-bought or homemade)
- Ricotta cheese
- Mixed berries
- Honey (optional)

Instructions:

1. Fill crepes with a mixture of ricotta cheese and mixed berries.
2. Drizzle with honey if desired.

Nutritional Information (per serving):

Calories: 220, Carbs: 30g, Protein: 8g, Fat: 8g, Fiber: 4g

Pumpkin Pie Chia Pudding:

Preparation Time: 10 minutes (plus chilling time)

Servings: 2

Ingredients:

- 1/4 cup chia seeds
- 1 cup unsweetened almond milk
- Pumpkin puree
- Pumpkin pie spice, stevia (optional)

Instructions:

1. Mix chia seeds, almond milk, pumpkin puree, pumpkin pie spice, and stevia.
2. Refrigerate until set.

Nutritional Information (per serving):

Calories: 180, Carbs: 20g, Protein: 6g, Fat: 9g, Fiber: 10g

Almond Flour Blueberry Muffins:

Cooking Time: 25 minutes

Servings: 6

Ingredients:

- 1 cup almond flour
- Eggs
- Unsweetened applesauce
- Blueberries
- Baking soda, vanilla extract

Instructions:

1. Mix almond flour, eggs, applesauce, blueberries, baking soda, and vanilla extract.
2. Bake until golden brown.

Nutritional Information (per serving):

Calories: 180, Carbs: 10g, Protein: 6g, Fat: 12g, Fiber: 3g

CHAPTER 6

BEVERAGES

Minty Green Tea Cooler:

Preparation Time: 10 minutes

Servings: 2

Ingredients:

- Green tea bags
- Fresh mint leaves
- Lemon slices
- Stevia (optional)

Instructions:

1. Brew green tea and let it cool.
2. Add fresh mint leaves, lemon slices, and stevia for sweetness.

Nutritional Information (per serving):

Calories: 5, Carbs: 1g, Protein: 0g, Fat: 0g, Fiber: 0g

Turmeric and Ginger Golden Milk:

Preparation Time: 15 minutes

Servings: 2

Ingredients:

- Almond milk
- Turmeric powder
- Fresh ginger, grated.
- Cinnamon, black pepper
- Honey (optional)

Instructions:

1. Heat almond milk with turmeric, ginger, cinnamon, and black pepper.
2. Sweeten with honey if desired.

Nutritional Information (per serving):

Calories: 60, Carbs: 8g, Protein: 1g, Fat: 3g, Fiber: 1g

Berry and Spinach Smoothie:

Preparation Time: 5 minutes

Servings: 1

Ingredients:

- Mixed berries (strawberries, blueberries)
- Spinach leaves
- Almond milk
- Protein powder (optional)

Instructions:

1. Blend berries, spinach, almond milk, and protein powder until smooth.
2. Adjust sweetness as needed.

Nutritional Information (per serving):

Calories: 120, Carbs: 15g, Protein: 5g, Fat: 5g, Fiber: 4g

Cucumber and Lemon Infused Water:

Preparation Time: 5 minutes

Servings: 2

Ingredients:

- Cucumber slices
- Lemon slices
- Fresh mint leaves
- Water

Instructions:

1. Combine cucumber slices, lemon slices, and mint leaves in a pitcher of water.
2. Refrigerate for refreshing infused water.

Nutritional Information (per serving):

Calories: 0, Carbs: 0g, Protein: 0g, Fat: 0g, Fiber: 0g

Iced Peppermint Chamomile Tea:

Preparation Time: 10 minutes

Servings: 2

Ingredients:

- Chamomile tea bags
- Peppermint tea bags
- Stevia (optional)
- Ice cubes

Instructions:

1. Brew chamomile and peppermint tea, let it cool.
2. Sweeten with stevia and serve over ice.

Nutritional Information (per serving):

Calories: 5, Carbs: 1g, Protein: 0g, Fat: 0g, Fiber: 0g

Coconut Water and Pineapple Smoothie:

Preparation Time: 5 minutes

Servings: 1

Ingredients:

- Coconut water
- Pineapple chunks
- Greek yogurt
- Ice cubes

Instructions:

1. Blend coconut water, pineapple chunks, and Greek yogurt with ice until smooth.
2. Serve immediately.

Nutritional Information (per serving):

Calories: 120, Carbs: 20g, Protein: 5g, Fat: 2g, Fiber: 2g

Matcha Green Tea Latte:

Preparation Time: 5 minutes

Servings: 1

Ingredients:

- Matcha green tea powder
- Almond milk
- Stevia (optional)

Instructions:

1. Whisk matcha powder with a small amount of hot water until dissolved.
2. Heat almond milk and pour over the matcha mixture. Sweeten with stevia.

Nutritional Information (per serving):

Calories: 30, Carbs: 2g, Protein: 1g, Fat: 2g, Fiber: 1g

Watermelon and Mint Agua Fresca:

Preparation Time: 15 minutes

Servings: 2

Ingredients:

- Watermelon cubes
- Fresh mint leaves
- Lime juice
- Water

Instructions:

1. Blend watermelon cubes, mint leaves, and lime juice until smooth.
2. Strain and dilute with water. Serve over ice.

Nutritional Information (per serving):

Calories: 60, Carbs: 15g, Protein: 1g, Fat: 0g, Fiber: 1g

Hibiscus Ginger Iced Tea:

Preparation Time: 10 minutes

Servings: 2

Ingredients:

- Hibiscus tea bags
- Fresh ginger, sliced.
- Stevia (optional)
- Ice cubes

Instructions:

1. Brew hibiscus tea with fresh ginger, let it cool.
2. Sweeten with stevia and serve over ice.

Nutritional Information (per serving):

Calories: 5, Carbs: 1g, Protein: 0g, Fat: 0g, Fiber: 0g

Raspberry and Basil Sparkling Water:

Preparation Time: 5 minutes

Servings: 2

Ingredients:

- Fresh raspberries
- Fresh basil leaves
- Sparkling water
- Lime slices

Instructions:

1. Muddle raspberries and basil in the bottom of a glass.
2. Fill the glass with sparkling water and add lime slices.

Nutritional Information (per serving):

Calories: 0, Carbs: 1g, Protein: 0g, Fat: 0g, Fiber: 1g

CHAPTER 7
14-DAY MEAL PLAN

Day 1:

- Breakfast: Baked Lemon Herb Chicken
- Lunch: Quinoa Salad with Veggies
- Dinner: Chickpea and Spinach Curry
- Snack: Greek Yogurt and Berry Parfait

Day 2:

- Breakfast: Vegetarian Lentil Soup
- Lunch: Turkey and Vegetable Stir-Fry with Brown Rice
- Dinner: Stuffed Bell Peppers with Quinoa and Black Beans
- Snack: Cucumber and Hummus Slices

Day 3:

- Breakfast: Grilled Salmon with Broccoli and Quinoa
- Lunch: Eggplant and Chickpea Curry
- Dinner: Spaghetti Squash with Turkey Bolognese
- Snack: Roasted Chickpeas

Day 4:

- Breakfast: Cauliflower Fried Rice with Shrimp
- Lunch: Lentil Soup with Mixed Greens Salad
- Dinner: Lemon Garlic Shrimp Zoodle Bowl
- Snack: Avocado and Tomato Salsa

Day 5:

- Breakfast: Baked Lemon Herb Chicken
- Lunch: Quinoa Salad with Veggies
- Dinner: Chickpea and Spinach Curry
- Snack: Greek Yogurt and Berry Parfait

Day 6:

- Breakfast: Vegetarian Lentil Soup
- Lunch: Turkey and Vegetable Stir-Fry with Brown Rice
- Dinner: Stuffed Bell Peppers with Quinoa and Black Beans
- Snack: Cucumber and Hummus Slices

Day 7:

- Breakfast: Grilled Salmon with Broccoli and Quinoa
- Lunch: Eggplant and Chickpea Curry
- Dinner: Spaghetti Squash with Turkey Bolognese
- Snack: Roasted Chickpeas

Day 8:

- Breakfast: Cauliflower Fried Rice with Shrimp
- Lunch: Lentil Soup with Mixed Greens Salad
- Dinner: Lemon Garlic Shrimp Zoodle Bowl
- Snack: Avocado and Tomato Salsa

Day 9:

- Breakfast: Chia Seed Pudding with Berries
- Lunch: Ricotta and Berry Stuffed Crepes
- Dinner: Turkey and Vegetable Stir-Fry with Brown Rice
- Snack: Greek Yogurt and Berry Parfait

Day 10:

- Breakfast: Dark Chocolate Avocado Mousse
- Lunch: Stuffed Bell Peppers with Quinoa and Black Beans
- Dinner: Eggplant and Chickpea Curry
- Snack: Cucumber and Hummus Slices

Day 11:

- Breakfast: Coconut Water and Pineapple Smoothie
- Lunch: Quinoa Salad with Veggies
- Dinner: Lemon Garlic Shrimp Zoodle Bowl
- Snack: Almond and Berry Smoothie

Day 12:

- Breakfast: Almond Flour Blueberry Muffins
- Lunch: Turkey and Vegetable Stir-Fry with Brown Rice
- Dinner: Chickpea and Spinach Curry
- Snack: Watermelon and Mint Agua Fresca

Day 13:

- Breakfast: Pumpkin Pie Chia Pudding
- Lunch: Grilled Salmon with Broccoli and Quinoa
- Dinner: Spaghetti Squash with Turkey Bolognese
- Snack: Raspberry and Basil Sparkling Water

Day 14:

- Breakfast: Iced Peppermint Chamomile Tea
- Lunch: Lentil Soup with Mixed Greens Salad
- Dinner: Cauliflower Fried Rice with Shrimp
- Snack: Almond and Berry Smoothie

CONCLUSION

As we reach the final pages of this cookbook, my heart swells with a mix of gratitude and anticipation. The journey we've taken together, you and I, is more than a mere exploration of recipes; it is a shared odyssey through the triumphs and challenges of living with PCOS. In the warmth of these culinary creations, I hope you've found not just nourishment for your body but also a comforting embrace for your spirit.

Reflect for a moment on the stories we've encountered—the journey of my dear friend Sophie and the countless women who, like her, sought solace in the alchemy of these recipes. Each meal, each bite, is a testament to the resilience of the human spirit and the transformative power of mindful, purposeful nourishment.

As you close this book, let the aroma of the recipes linger in your kitchen, carrying with it the promise of possibility. This is not a farewell; it's an invitation to make these recipes a part of your daily ritual, a celebration of self-love and well-being. The journey towards wellness is ongoing, and with each dish, you are writing a new chapter in your own story of triumph.

Consider this: the spices that danced on your taste buds, the colors that adorned your plate, and the nutrients that fueled your body—they are not just ingredients; they are the building blocks of a healthier, more vibrant you. In each recipe, I've poured not just my knowledge as a dietician but also my compassion as a friend who understands the challenges you face.

As you navigate the world beyond these pages, remember that you are not alone. The community of women embracing these recipes as a lifeline continues to grow, and their collective strength is a testament to the potential for healing that resides within each one of us. Share your journey, your victories, and your discoveries. Let the ripple effect of wellness touch the lives of those around you, just as it has touched yours.

And so, with a heart brimming with hope, I extend my deepest gratitude for allowing me to be a part of your wellness journey. As you savor the last morsel of inspiration within these pages, know that the power to transform your life lies not just in the recipes but in the love and care you extend to yourself. May your days be filled with joy, your body with vitality, and your spirit with the unwavering belief that you are deserving of a life beautifully nourished.

Here's to you, to the stories yet to unfold, and to the delicious journey that lies ahead. Embrace it with open arms, savor each moment, and relish the magic that happens when food becomes not just sustenance but a celebration of life. Until we meet again, be well, be nourished, and most importantly, be kind to yourself.

BONUS

EXERCISE AND LIFESTYLE

Exercise plays a crucial role in managing PCOS (Polycystic Ovary Syndrome) and promoting overall well-being. Here are some key reasons why exercise is important for individuals with PCOS:

Improved Insulin Sensitivity:

Regular exercise enhances insulin sensitivity, reducing the risk of insulin resistance in individuals with PCOS. This is crucial for managing blood sugar levels effectively.

Weight Management:

Exercise aids in weight management, which is significant for women with PCOS, as excess weight can worsen symptoms and hormonal imbalances, contributing to insulin resistance.

Hormonal Regulation:

Physical activity plays a role in regulating hormones, including insulin, cortisol, and reproductive hormones. This regulation can help restore menstrual regularity and improve fertility.

Metabolic Health:

Engaging in physical activity positively impacts lipid profiles and reduces cardiovascular risk factors, addressing metabolic concerns often associated with PCOS.

Stress Reduction:

Exercise is a natural stress reliever. Managing stress is crucial for individuals with PCOS, as elevated stress levels can exacerbate symptoms. Regular exercise helps reduce cortisol levels and improves overall mental well-being.

Improved Mood and Energy Levels:

The release of endorphins during exercise enhances mood and alleviates symptoms of anxiety and depression often experienced by individuals with PCOS.

Enhanced Fertility:

For those seeking to conceive, exercise can improve fertility by promoting hormonal balance and optimizing overall health, including a healthy body weight.

Types of Exercise for PCOS:

Aerobic Exercise:

Activities like brisk walking, jogging, cycling, and swimming improve cardiovascular health, boost metabolism, and aid in weight management.

Strength Training:

Resistance training with weights or resistance bands helps build lean muscle mass, enhance metabolism, and improve overall body composition.

Yoga:

Combining physical postures, breath control, and meditation, yoga is beneficial for reducing stress, improving flexibility, and promoting relaxation.

High-Intensity Interval Training (HIIT):

HIIT involves short bursts of intense exercise followed by periods of rest. It is effective for improving insulin sensitivity and burning calories.

Pilates:

Focused on core strength, flexibility, and overall body conditioning, Pilates is helpful for improving posture and strength.

Dance Workouts:

Zumba or dance aerobics provide a fun way to stay active, offering cardiovascular benefits while making exercise enjoyable.

Mind-Body Exercises:

Tai Chi or Qigong combines movement, meditation, and breathing techniques, promoting relaxation and stress reduction.

Stress Management Techniques:

Mindfulness Meditation:

Mindfulness meditation involves focusing on the present moment, reducing stress and promoting mental well-being.

Deep Breathing Exercises:

Practicing deep breathing exercises, such as diaphragmatic breathing, activates the body's relaxation response, reducing stress.

Progressive Muscle Relaxation (PMR):

PMR involves systematically tensing and relaxing muscle groups, promoting physical and mental relaxation.

Biofeedback:

Biofeedback techniques help individuals gain awareness and control over physiological functions, aiding in stress management.

Regular Relaxation Time:

Dedicate time daily to activities that bring joy and relaxation, promoting mental well-being.

Social Support:

Building a strong support system provides emotional support during stressful times, improving overall resilience.

Counseling or Therapy:

Professional counseling or therapy offers valuable tools and coping mechanisms for managing stress and improving mental health.

Incorporating a combination of these stress management techniques and a personalized exercise plan can contribute to holistic well-being for individuals with PCOS.